THE BELL'S BOOK

THE BELL'S BOOK

AN ESSENTIAL GUIDE TO BELL'S PALSY AND HOW TO TAKE BACK YOUR SMILE

DR. WILLIAM K. LAWRENCE

PARAMOUNT EDUCATION

The Bell's Book
William K. Lawrence © 2020
© 2022 updates
All rights reserved
ISBN: 978-1-7356871-0-0

Paramount Education Press
Washington D.C., United States

Cover concept: JL

Cover Designer:
Nojus Modestas Jankevičius

Disclaimer:

This book is meant to be support for you in this difficult time. The book is not a replacement for medical treatment, nor is it written by a medical doctor who is treating you for this ailment.

FOR ALL THOSE WHO HAVE FELT
THE TAKING OF THEIR SMILE

CONTENTS

WARNING

Before you read another paragraph, get to your doctor's office or emergency room if you haven't been there yet. Deferring the routine steroids has been found to delay and even damage your chances of full recovery. If a doctor has not diagnosed you with Bell's Palsy, be sure a medical professional has ruled it out for sure. A misdiagnosis leads to deferral of treatment, which means less chance of recovery.

THE SYMPTOMS:

- Paralysis on one side of the face from the forehead down to the jawline with the inability to move the affected side, which results in drooping

- Numbness on the lips, which affects speech

- Loss of taste

- Pain on the cheek and back of the head behind the ear

- Strange hearing imbalance on the affected side; sometimes hyper-sensitive to sounds; sometimes muffled echo-like feeling similar to having swimmer's ear

- Inability to fully close the eye on the affected side, which results in excessive tearing and light sensitivity

You are likely to have all of these listed symptoms, sometimes all at once for true Bell's Palsy. This disorder is no walk in the park. It will mess with you in multiple ways, so you'll want to stay strong through this and call on your loved ones for support.

If you have any numbness below your jaw in the affected side, go to the emergency room or call 911. Your arms and legs should not be affected by a true case of Bell's Palsy. Loss of feeling or the inability to walk or balance one or both of your arms are signs of a stroke. If the numbness is isolated to your face, there is a great chance you have Bell's Palsy.

Bell's Palsy comes on suddenly usually upon waking up. If you have slowly degenerated into facial paralysis, there is more reason to rush to your neurologist or ER because it is most certainly another matter. True Bell's is not a reason to panic.

Likely and hopefully, you're now reading this paperback book days later as a survivor of only Bell's Palsy.

INTRODUCTION

So you've woken up and your face is crooked and your smile is missing. You might not have discovered it until you went to eat breakfast and the food leaked out the side of your mouth. Or maybe you went to splash water on your face upon waking, only to feel something strange on one side, to look up and find half your face has slid off to the south. Your mouth hangs on one side. There's an odd numbness. You struggle to speak.

Before getting to your primary doctor or the ER, you considered the possibility that you were having a stroke (which is nothing to fool around with)— only to realize the numbness was isolated to your face, and the rest of your body was safely and fully functional.

Once you safely ruled out a stroke, hopefully you still got to the doctor relatively quick. Any delay in the usage of steroids and anti-viral medication will lead to a delay in healing. You should be prescribed an oral corticosteroid drug, such as prednisone, as well as an anti-viral medication.

Once you've been properly diagnosed and prescribed medication, you are on your way to coping with a disorder known as Bell's Palsy.

Push for the correct diagnosis. According to a *BBC* report, 19% of patients dealt with a misdiagnosis that stunted their recovery. That's just not acceptable.

Before experiencing this disorder firsthand, you might have thought Bell's Palsy was some effect of not taking care of yourself. Maybe you thought it was a birth defect. Sometimes it is confused with cerebral palsy. But Bell's is none of those. Perfectly healthy people, mostly in their late teens to late thirties, wake up with this disorder. It is a condition that comes out of nowhere and can strike anyone at anytime. This book will discuss the highlights in the medical literature and equip you with lifestyle recommendations to assist you with your recovery in the quickest way possible.

When I suddenly woke up with this odd disorder, I went right to Google. My brother in law Andy had woken up with Bell's only a year earlier, so I was somewhat familiar with the condition, but certainly not prepared for it. I really had had no idea what Andy had gone through; no one really had. And that's one thing you need to realize early on: unless someone else has had this, it's going to be difficult for anyone else to grasp the internal struggles you will go through.

The good news is this disorder is not permanent or dangerous, most of the time. "Things could always be worse" became my motto.

One of the first things many of you will do when you get home from the doctor's office with that first diagnosis is jump onto an Internet search. Google is going to deliver over 1.1 million results. Many of the medical organizations with .org websites are going to repeat the same information over and over, though some sites will give you one or two new tidbits to consider. Other .com and .net websites provide opinions and theories that aren't always credible. Some people express some pretty wild ideas on their blogs and sites.

Some websites even recommended outdated procedures like taping your eye shut at night, which hasn't been recommended in decades! Be careful whom you listen to on the Internet.

The same frustration occurred when I went to find books on the subject. Some of the books are overdone and confusing with medical jargon, some are very misleading and incomplete, and some books promote just one approach. For example, there is no reason you need to read hundreds of pages to get down to the basics of recovering from this disorder. That's an author or publisher stretching the page count so they can meet an industry standard, and charge you more. There's also no reason to read an entire book that just repeats something found in every web reference to the disorder. These are the reasons why I wrote this book. The Bell's Book will save you time, money, and energy. You will need those for your healing.

I am fortunate to be in the education field and have access to medical journals in the scholarly databases. After a broad Internet search, I moved to the deeper peer reviewed journal articles for more specific and credible information. I wanted to find out what the most recent studies were showing. The journals discussed treatments and findings not available to the general public on those .org or .gov websites and certainly not on the less credible .com and .net sites. I then went and read several older studies for a sense of the history. International perspectives found in medical journals from around the world were also a tremendous help.

What I've done in this brief book is compile the most interesting and helpful information on the condition. This is not an unnecessarily detailed (and exhausting) book that only doctors and scientists can read. This is a book meant for the average person to understand and benefit from. Occasionally, there is no other way around using a medical term, but I've made an effort to simplify this book to make it readable for more people. Return to it when you need and use it as a guide through your recovery.

I am an educator and researcher. I am experienced with the condition. But I am not your medical doctor, so keep in mind that I'm relaying expert information, statistics, and facts from outside credible primary research studies and secondary sources in addition to my firsthand observation. I am also translating all of this into language everyone can make sense of. I urge you to still visit your primary care doctor and neurologist. In the chapter on treatment, I share what helped me. All of these approaches have been found to help many others as well, but keep in mind everyone's journey is different. How we heal and what approaches we emphasize are going to depend on our individual needs, but what we have in common is a mutual path to recovery.

In your initial Google search, you certainly encountered thousands of visuals. People with crooked smiles. People with one eye seeming to bulge while the other one barely opens. Twisted faces. Droopy faces. Hideous versions of what we all once were. Some of these photographs can be frightening. Some will make you feel better if your case isn't as severe. Seeing pictures of people tracking the condition week by week can also provide hope since most of you can expect a full or near full recovery.

There's no doubt. You've been hit with a lousy condition, and there may be some scary moments and social struggles, but you can beat this. Think of yourself as chosen, cursed, or blessed, but know that there will be people in that neurologist's office who will not be recovering from their injuries or disease. You have hope. Lots of it.

Why me? Why now? What can I do about it? Read on for a brief education on the condition or feel free to jump around to different chapters, as you need them. My own story is at the end if you prefer to start there, or skip to the treatment chapter to get started on your recovery. But keep in mind that I've kept everything brief and simple, so working through in the provided sequence will not be too taxing. The fewer words you have to weed through, the more you can focus on your recovery and the quicker you will heal.

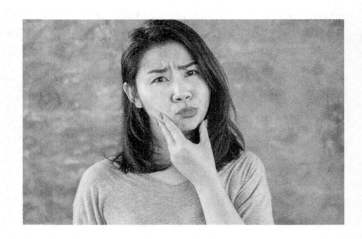

WHAT IS BELL'S PALSY?

Bell's Palsy is a mysterious condition that usually paralyzes one side of the face. Thankfully, there are very few cases where people are struck with both sides of the face all at once. Bell's Palsy is idiopathic, which means doctors and scientists have no idea why it happens. They know the nerve line in your face is damaged due to inflammation, but they don't know exactly why it happens.

Researchers believe the inflammation is caused by injury or virus, but they have not been able to isolate the viral DNA in a biopsy. The strongest suspect is the human herpes virus, which lies dormant in our nervous system undetected for decades.

History

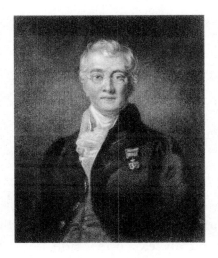

The condition is named after 19th century Scottish doctor Sir Charles Bell (see above) who studied the anatomy of the facial nerve and unilateral facial palsy. Dr. Bell (1774-1842) discovered the difference between sensory nerves and motor nerves in the spinal cord and then made the connection between the seventh cranial nerve and facial palsy in his 1821 paper *On the Nerves: Giving an Account of some Experiments on Their Structure and Functions, Which Lead to a New Arrangement of the System.* Bell also wrote *Essays on The Anatomy of Expression in Painting* in 1806. Bell was also quite an illustrator. This is Plate II from Charles Bell's *Anatomy and Philosophy of Expression* (1844, third edition) as found in the public domain:

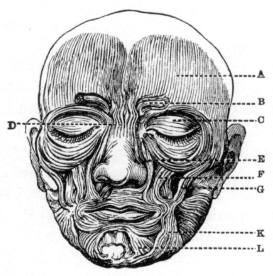

Fɪɢ. 1.—Diagram of the muscles of the face, from Sir C. Bell.

Bell's Palsy has been around forever. The ancient thinkers of Egypt, Greece, Rome, and native cultures documented and acknowledged the disorder. The early Greek Physician and "father of medicine" Hippocrates (5th Century BCE) made references to facial nerve disorders: "Distortions of the face, if they coincide with no other disorder of the body, quickly cease, either spontaneously or as the result of treatment. Otherwise there is paralysis." Areteaus (1st century CE) described paralysis, including parts of the face: "Wherefore, the parts are sometimes paralyzed singly, as one eye-brow..."

An early comprehensive description of the disorder was completed by 9th-century Persian physician Abu Bakr Muhammad ibn Zakariya Razi (865–925 CE). Razi described bilateral facial palsy: "I have seen a man who...was affected by a type of facial distortion in which his face was not crooked, but one of his eyes he could barely close...and when drinking, water would flow from his mouth." Razi's book *al-Hawi* included a section on the disorder and was first translated into Latin in 1279. Even though it was published in Europe in 1468, it was never translated into English and was not read widely by those across Europe.

Abu al-Hasan Ali ibn Sahl Rabban al-Tabari (838–870 CE) was another Persian physician who wrote of the condition: "If half of the face becomes paralyzed, it will be drawn to the healthy side, because the muscles that are healthy are strong, and will pull the paralyzed muscles toward itself."

Other early physicians such as Cornelis van der Wiel (1620-1702), James Douglas (1675-1742), Nicolaus A. Friedreich (1761-1836), and Evert Jan Thomassen à Thuessink (1762-1832) studied and wrote about facial palsy. Van der Wiel described a female patient with a "twisting of the mouth" that was cured after a few weeks. Friedreich wrote an extensive thesis on the matter in 1797 in Germany and described the condition as Rheumatic Facial Paralysis. Richard Powell observed, studied, and reported the onset and recovery in 1813. One of the oldest research papers in modern databases dates back to 1927.

Theories

In the modern age of medicine in the twentieth century, doctors hypothesized about Bell's Palsy. Early conclusions seem to be more speculative. By 1945, some researchers believed dental infections caused Bell's Palsy, which seems reasonable because dental infections can affect your face, and dental surgeons often avoid impacted wisdom tooth extractions on people older than forty due to risk of nerve damage. But this theory never really developed with any evidence.

The herpes virus theory has held up much better through the years. There are at least nine herpes viruses that infect humans. Five types are so common that at least 90% of adults have been infected with at least one, as pointed out by Wald and Corey.

In 1941, researchers in clinical observations tied Bell's Palsy to herpes varicella zoster, which produces chickenpox and shingles. The medical research was still too limited to prove anything. One newer study in Brazil in 2010 involving 171 participants found only two Bell's patients (1.7%) to have varicella zoster virus (VZV) in their saliva samples. Just because they didn't find it, doesn't mean it wasn't there, but 2 out of 171 is awfully low.

In 1971, Dr. David McCormick argued that a different type of herpes virus known as simplex (HSV) was a cause of Bell's. Herpes simplex virus was found in 21.9% of cases in a 1999 medical study by Chakravarti et al. In a separate reactivation group, the number was closer to 50%. However, these percentages are just not high enough to be considered a proven cause. The researchers pointed out that they only tested for type 1 and acknowledged that perhaps there are different causes.

In a 1996 paper, Murakami et al. had concluded that herpes simplex type 1 was the cause of Bell's Palsy. HSV was detected in 11 of 14 patients (79%) with Bell's Palsy, but the study had an extremely small sample size of subjects, which casts doubt on the claim. The researchers also did not detect HSV in patients with the more serious Ramsay-Hunt syndrome. According to Sweeney et al., herpes zoster virus has been found more definitively to cause Ramsay-Hunt Syndrome, which causes similar but more extreme symptoms.

In 2001, Takahasahi et al. were able to induce facial palsy in mice during animal testing using the herpes simplex virus. However, only 58% of the mice developed facial palsy. Even if animal testing was reliable for this, which it is not, it's clearly still not enough to prove that the herpes simplex virus alone causes Bell's Palsy.

Speaking of animals, they too are victims of facial palsy. According to Varejao et al., the most common form of facial paralysis in dogs is idiopathic. Other causes of facial paralysis in nonhuman animals have been linked to hypothyroidism, ear infection, trauma, and lesions, according to William Thomas, DVM.

Facial palsy has been observed in cats, dogs, horses, and other mammals.

In 2020, some COVID-19 patients developed facial paralysis. One study by Dr. Lima et al. reported eight COVID-19 patients with facial palsy. Seven of them were female, four of them were in their thirties, and five of them showed complete recovery. Half were affected on the left side of the face and half on the right side. This finding seems to go along well with the viral theory, but there are two major problems. Why did most COVID-19 patients not develop facial palsy? Even further, why do Bell's Palsy patients fail to show any other viral symptoms?

Researchers have moved closer to identifying a virus as a secondary cause, (enough that they will prescribe an anti-viral drug), but they are still unable to isolate any virus in a biopsy from patients for final confirmation. Regardless of which virus, the majority of people with viruses do not develop facial palsy. It may be that Bell's Palsy is caused by multiple factors and driven by underlying viral activity, but no one virus may be the cause.

There has also been a belief in the potential for Bell's Palsy to spread like a contagious virus, but there is no conclusive evidence.

Reaves et al. discovered a cluster in 2011 with three cases of Bell's Palsy in one office building, which is an amazing coincidence for such a rare disorder. But they were ultimately unable to pinpoint a causal connection.

While vaccines are critical to human health (and all recommended vaccines should be completed, at least on an alternative schedule), there have been some very rare findings linking them to Bell's Palsy. A Switzerland study by Mutsch et al. discovered that an intranasal vaccine was found to increase the risk of Bell's Palsy. A Swedish study by Bardage et al. found that relative risks were increased for Bell's Palsy after vaccination for influenza A. Another study by Tseng et al. published in *Pediatrics* argued an association between occurrence of Bell's Palsy and Meningococcal conjugate vaccination. Hepatitis B vaccination was also thought to be a rare cause of Bell's, according to Dr. Alp et al. as published in the *Journal of Health and Popular Nutrition.* Keep in mind, these rare results have not been duplicated.

During the height of the 2020 pandemic, conspiracy theories about the Covid vaccine were spread on the internet. However, Bell's Palsy among vaccine recipients is about the same as in the general population, which means you have the same chance of developing the disorder after receiving the vaccine as you do before getting the vaccine, as reported by Cassie Drumm for the Jefferson Facial Nerve Center. The argument that the vaccine causes Bell's Palsy is a false cause logic fallacy. B is not caused by A just because it comes after it. We'll revisit these beliefs later in the book.

Stress is another unconfirmed cause for Bell's Palsy. Many experts suspect that stress can trigger a virus, which then causes the inflammation. In the UK where there is a one in sixty lifetime risk of developing Bell's Palsy, a recent survey of 421 patients revealed that more than half had suffered from anxiety and depression, according to the UK Facial Palsy Organization. We know that stress takes its toll on your immune system. We know a lowered immune system leads to all kinds of ailments, so perhaps stress is one of the roots.

Although there have been documented cases of Bell's across multiple generations of family, it has also not been proven to be hereditary. In 2021, Skuladottir et al. argued for a genetic link after finding the first association between Bell's Palsy and sequence variant rs9357446-

A. Yet the researchers could not conclude with confidence. They ultimately fell back on the virus theory and acknowledged that Bell's is still idiopathic. However, perhaps this is just the beginning of finding both a genetic source and treatment.

Have all these various conflicting theories confused you yet? Bell's Palsy is surely one of the most argued and mysterious disorders. In Eastern medicine, the Chinese refer to Bell's Palsy as a wind stroke and believe both internal and external "winds" disrupt the body's balance. Maybe they're right too. Even with all these years of research, it seems we do not know much more about the cause than Charles Bell did in 1821.

The Facts

Here's what we do know. The face has twelve cranial nerves. The nerve that is affected when you have Bell's is the seventh cranial nerve, sometimes listed as CNVII. This 7th cranial nerve is responsible for facial movement. This nerve affects the stapedius muscle of the middle ear, which is why you are probably having strange sensations in the ear on the affected side. The 7th cranial nerve also affects taste, which is why you might have a loss of taste. The nerve travels through a narrow, bony canal in the skull. Bell's Palsy happens when there is a disruption to that nerve, which causes an interruption in the communication between the brain and the nerve.

General facial paralysis is caused by multiple factors that impact the area and lead to inflammation of the nerve. Trauma to the head and face is one cause. Misplaced dental anesthetic can cause facial paralysis, though the effects should dissipate quickly. A tumor could also be the cause. Lower motor neuron lesions can result in palsy after damaging the cranial nerve, which can disturb speech, swallowing, taste, and the tongue muscle. Bacterial infections such as Lyme disease have also been found to cause facial paralysis.

Bell's Palsy has been found to have a higher incidence in pregnant women and people with diabetes. The more elevated the glycated hemoglobin level, the more severe the facial palsy. Risk factors for Bell's Palsy include pregnancy, preeclampsia, diabetes, and hypertension. Pregnant women who develop Bell's Palsy should be screened for pre-eclampsia.

Idiopathic facial palsy (true Bell's Palsy) is the most common listed "cause" while the second most common cause of facial palsy is cerebro vascular accident. A diagnosis of Bell's Palsy is defined as vascular congestion and entrapment neuropathy resulting from inflammation, edema, and strangulation. In other words, something pressed on the nerve and damaged it. The problem is experts cannot determine what exactly leads to those causes. The process is clear, but the cause remains an enigma. The good news is true Bell's Palsy is a lot less to worry about than facial palsy caused by other factors.

Diagnosis

Your neurologist will likely use the House-Brackmann scale to determine the severity of your case. The House-Brackmann scale is an evaluation system developed in 1985 by Dr. John W. House and Dr. Derald Brackmann. One point is assigned for every 0.25 cm of motion for both eyebrow and mouth movement, with a maximum of 1 cm. The scale is not the only tool used for continuing treatment, but it is standard in the initial evaluation.

HOUSE-BRACKMANN SCALE

Grade I: Normal

Grade II: Slight facial weakness or other mild dysfunction. Normal tone and symmetry at rest. Complete closure of the eye without effort. Slight asymmetry of the mouth when facial movements occur.

Grade III: Moderate dysfunction; these patients generally do not display any noticeable facial weakness, they maintain complete eye closure and good forehead movement with effort.

Grade IV: Moderate severe dysfunction. Obvious facial weakness. Asymmetrical mouth movement. No forehead movement. Incomplete eye closure.

Grade V: Severe dysfunction. Motion is barely perceptible. Slight mouth movement. No forehead movement. The eye is unable to close. Function is at 1-25%.

Grade VI: Total paralysis. No facial motion.

Numbers

International research studies reveal five important distinctions:
1. Bell's is 60-75% of all cases of facial palsy.
2. There are more cases during colder winter months and less during warmer months.
3. The right side of the face is more common.
4. Men are slightly more likely to get Bell's.
5. 85% of people who are diagnosed with Bell's Palsy recover within a few months.

Bell's Palsy is a global disease that can strike anyone anywhere. An estimated one million people are struck with Bell's every year around the world and will share your struggle. Between 12,400 and 24,800 will get Bell's in the UK each year. In Germany, there are between 7 and 40 cases per 100,000. In Spain, there are between 11 and 40 cases per 100,000 each year on average, though the numbers have been as high as 240 per 100,000. Although it only strikes 1 in 65 in the United States, that's still about 40,000 Americans every year. The highest incidence found to date was in Seckori, Japan in 1986, and the lowest was found in Sweden in 1971.

While researchers have pointed to no geographic difference in the incidence of Bell's Palsy, many countries have poor reporting or no reporting at all, so improved international efforts are needed for tracking this disorder. Keep in mind, there is no place in the world that hasn't had cases of Bell's Palsy. The following table contains a sampling of reported data based on averages of the population. There is a sure margin of error due to reporting flaws and victims who sadly do not or cannot seek treatment.

International snapshot:

Nation	Out of 100,000 people
Germany	7-40
Spain	11-40
Australia	11-40
U.S.	15-23
Sudan	15-30
China	20-30
India	25
Japan	30
Italy	53

Most population studies generally show an annual incidence of 15–30 cases per 100,000 of the population. Some nations see higher numbers some years, so the table is only a snapshot of a recent available year. I could find no study that compared and contrasted years in geographic locations, and one reason might be poor reporting even in the best of developed nations. I would recommend future studies to examine contrasts and locations.

If we take the average percentage into account, we're talking about nearly 450,000 people afflicted with Bell's Palsy just in China and India alone each year. Those two countries see almost half of the 1,170,000 people around the globe who will wake up with a paralyzed face from Bell's Palsy every year!

A major Nigerian study published in *African Health Sciences*, revealed age 20-34 as the biggest group to wake up with facial palsy at 40.3%. Age 0-12 and 13-19 each had just 6.7%. The study found that "businessmen" had the largest incidence with over 30% more chance of developing facial palsy than medical professionals. Although just 39% of facial palsy cases in this study were true idiopathic Bell's Palsy, it was still the single biggest cause.

Other studies have identified peak incidence in our forties, but a portion of patients are in their twenties. The disease can strike teenagers and children on occasion too. Most recover quite quickly without any permanent mark. One study evaluated 170 children over a 17-year period and found that Bell's Palsy accounted for 42% of the facial nerve paralyses versus tumors at 2%.

Despite how awful this seems, if you or your child have woken up with this disorder, the numbers are in your favor. True Bell's Palsy is no danger, but that's why it is so important to rule out other conditions that cause facial palsy. Over 90% will recover quite well from Bell's Palsy. Others will need to work at it a little more. In fact, based on what I've seen, no one will slide through this condition and recover without putting in some effort.

Stay strong!

THE ANATOMY OF A SMILE

What is a smile? What makes a smile happen? People take the smile for granted. It's a simple smile, they think. How hard can it be? But there are many complex physiological steps to make a smile happen on your face.

The face has twelve cranial nerves. The nerve that is affected when you have Bell's is the seventh cranial nerve, sometimes listed as CNVII. The seventh cranial nerve exits the cerebral cortex and emerges from your skull just in front of your ears. It then splits into five primary branches: temporal, zygomatic, buccal, mandibular, and cervical. The 43 muscles in your face are completely useless without these nerves.

The seventh cranial nerve is responsible for facial movement. This nerve also affects the ears and tongue, so someone with Bell's will often have hearing and taste issues. The CNVII travels through a narrow, bony canal in the skull. Bell's Palsy happens when there is a disruption to that nerve, which causes an interruption in the communication between the brain and the nerve.

The Zygomatic Major is the muscle of facial expression, which draws the angle of the mouth superiorly and posteriorly to allow one to smile. Like all muscles of facial expression, the Zygomatic Major is innervated by the facial nerve (the seventh cranial nerve), more specifically, the buccal and zygomatic branches of the facial nerve. Over 70% of the subjects in one study by Penn et al. were able to perceive a smile with only 40% function of the unilateral paralyzed Zygomaticus Major. Without a contraction of the Zygomatic Major and the levator anguli oris, you cannot produce a noticeable smile.

The Zygomatic Major (colored in bright red in the diagram on the following page) is your smile muscle.

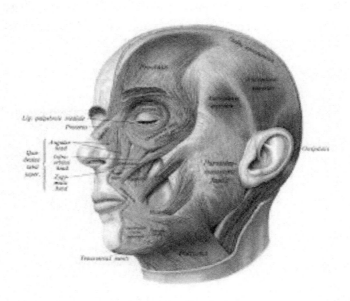

Zygomaticus Major Muscle

From Sobotta, in the Public Domain

As you can observe in the diagram below, the anatomy of the face is quite complicated! This is an anatomical illustration by Hermann Braus from the 1921 German edition of Anatomie des Menschen: ein Lehrbuch für Studierende und Ärzte with Latin terminology. This shows the many facial muscles we rely on to make expressions.

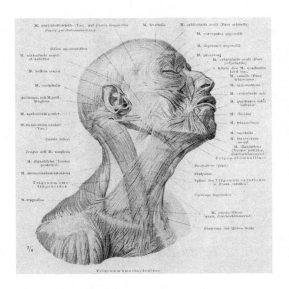

Face Muscles

From Braus, in the Public Domain

The nerves in your face are like a web that crawls underneath the surface of your skin. If you could pinch just one of these nerves, you will have loss of muscle and/or pain. The following visual demonstrates the side view of the facial nerve to show how much of your face it covers. Bell's Palsy happens when the nerve is damaged prior to branching out, just as it exits the ear area into the cheek.

The Facial Nerve

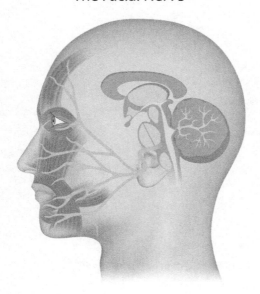

It all starts in the brain. Note the green facial nerve toward the bottom middle of this diagram. Your facial movements start with that little nerve. That's why the neurologist is your doctor of choice for this condition.

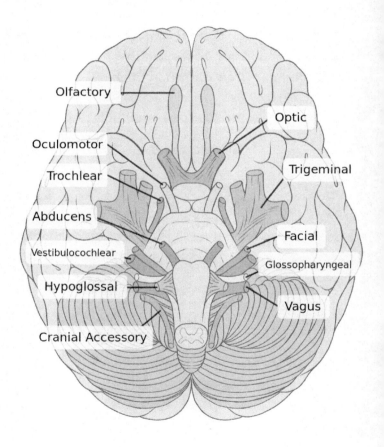

Medical Illustration: Patrick Lynch

The below photograph is a great illustration of someone with Bell's Palsy anywhere between week two and six. The man is smiling to the best of his ability. His right side is normal, but his left side is frozen in place. He does not have the severe droop some victims get, but he might also be a week or two beyond that initial phase, likely after a steroid treatment, which stabilizes the face. Notice the lost facial creases on the affected left side. While his left brow is not showing too much of a difference, you will notice the left eye is slightly enlarged; this is due to the eye on the affected side being unable to fully close or blink.

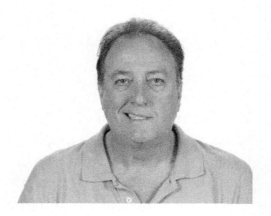

The woman below has a noticeably higher brow on the left affected side. The eye on the paralyzed side is essentially forced open and will appear bigger. Most have a strong enough case of Bell's that the paralysis runs higher up the face, which will also affect the ability to move the eyebrow or wrinkle the forehead.

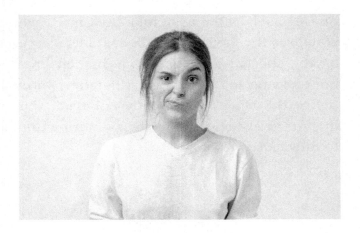

The human face is a marvelous creation. The face handles all five senses and enables us to communicate and eat. It's amazing that a boxer can take such hits (not without permanent damage of course), yet a whole side of the face is instantly shut down overnight by an unconfirmed stress on one little nerve.

THE SOCIOLOGY OF THE SMILE

The human smile is complicated. The result of Bell's Palsy, or lack of a smile, has huge sociological and psychological effects on the individual and the many people around that person. In his book *A Brief History of the Smile* Angus Trumble defines the smile:

> Of course, the smile is more than a chemical reaction, a series of muscular contractions, or a mechanism. It is a highly sophisticated concept, an expression of emotions, a mode of communication, a beacon of desire, a ritual—an occasion, in other words, of intense psychological, anthropological, and social interest, the product of acute observation, cognition, and interpretation. (p. 56)

Facial expressions are invaluable. A smile lets everyone know you are warm and safe and friendly. The frown lets everyone know you are dissatisfied. The smile is an expression of pleasure to people in the United States, but people in Russia consider publicly smiling at strangers to be unusual and even suspicious behavior. Levine and Adelman point out in their book *Beyond Language*:

> Some Russians believe that Americans smile in the wrong places; some Americans believe that Russians don't smile enough. In Southeast Asian cultures, a smile is frequently used to cover emotional pain or embarrassment. Vietnamese people may tell the sad story of how they had to leave their country but end the story with a smile.

In some parts of Asia, people may smile when they are embarrassed or in emotional pain. It's a coping mechanism, much the way someone might laugh in a moment of discomfort. It does not mean they are laughing because anything is funny.

Levine and Adelman also caution that we should not attempt to "read" people by their facial expressions. Yet how many times do we hear "a person must have committed a heinous crime because they looked like they were guilty because their face either showed guilt or a lack of empathy"? I can bet there are people in prison right now wrongfully convicted because they *looked* like they were guilty.

Sociologists have warned not to rely on facial analysis in criminal cases, with the consideration that everyone shows their emotions differently.

We know that culture, even local personal culture, differs. We know that people show or don't show their emotions and grief in radically different ways. We also know that physical displays are not at all reliable. All of this is because we are individuals with differing experience, culture, personality, types of intelligence, and patterns of thinking. We use our faces, yet they can be very deceiving.

Just ask any person with Bell's Palsy who is smiling inside but can't show that smile!

The smile may have evolved differently among different species, especially among humans. Primatologist Signe Preuschoft traced the smile back across 30 million years of evolution to a "fear grin" which originated with monkeys and apes who often used slightly clenched teeth to let predators know they were harmless. To this day the Barbary Macaque uses what might be considered the ancestor of our smile. If you don't think animals smile too, do a quick Google search.

The Smile in Pop Culture

Angus Trumble's book *A Brief History of the Smile* is a great read that spent months as a bedside book on my nightstand. After the basic descriptions, observations, and analysis of the smile, Trumble focuses a good portion of his book on art history. If you want to explore the smile in art, certainly check out that book next.

One thing Trumble does not get into— the many songs that feature the word smile in the title. There are hundreds of songs from multiple genres that feature the word smile in it. From pop, hip hop, rock, to country, there are hundreds of songs with "smile" in the title. Some of the popular artists who dedicated a song to the smile include Louis Armstrong, Maisie Peters, Mary J. Blige, Sarah Vaughan,

Barbara Streisand, Bad English, Nat King Cole, Fats Domino, Alanis Morrissette, Avril Lavigne, Michael Jackson, Julian Lennon, Hall & Oates, Taylor Swift, Dusty Springfield, Durand Jones and the Indications, David Gilmour, Pearl Jam, Weezer, Coldplay, The Killers, Everclear, Red Hot Chili Peppers, Cheap Trick, Barry Manilow, Usher, Stevie Wonder, Uncle Kracker, and so many more. The smile is so well represented in music that I was able to compile a Spotify playlist of over thirteen hours of songs with the word "smile" in the title!

Think about where else you see the smile around. There are hundreds of fictional books that carry the word smile in their titles. There are hundreds of films as well. Don't forget the evil smile perfected by so many actors playing villains in films.

What distinguishes the difference between a loving smile and a devious one? You might see the wild in a villain's eyes while they're smiling, which gives away their intent. But obviously looks can also be deceiving at first glance. Sometimes the character who looks unhappy is the hero and protagonist. Sometimes a smiley character can be made into a villain as in *The Joker,* who also has a problem with laughing.

The human smile is also well celebrated and used in advertising. The smile appeals to us and makes us feel accepted and comfortable. T-shirt companies like *Life is Good* use smiling cartoon characters. American Harvey Ball created the yellow and black smiley face graphic in 1963 that would go on to be an iconic cultural symbol. He later founded the World Smile Foundation and World Smile Day on the first Friday of October. Another version of the smiley face was created in 1971 by Franklin Loufrani and would be created into the Smiley company, which later created the internet emoticons we all know and use today.

Like laughter, smiling is healthy and contagious too. But what if that smile is taken by sadness or temporary grief? What if that smile is taken by long-term depression? For those folks, it's a matter of time, therapy, or medication to get their smiles back. A smile equals health.

But what if a disorder like Bell's Palsy steals that smile? The next chapter gives you what you need to fight back and take back your smile.

TREATMENT AND RECOVERY

Bell's Palsy should be treated aggressively with multiple approaches. Since it affects everyone in a different way, you will want to try as many treatments as possible. Do not expect an immediate cure. There is none. There is no magic pill. There is no quick surgical procedure. There is no treatment that will return you to your previous state overnight.

You must be active in your healing. Slow progress is often the result of someone expecting this disorder to get better on its own. You must try everything possible. Other than the initial steroid and anti-viral, there isn't much more your primary doctor can do for you. Even the neurologist is limited, and surgery to the nerve is only a long-term option for those whose symptoms persist, and even then the results are mixed. You've already taken the first step to healing by reading this book and becoming informed on the condition. Keep at it!

Something you probably found when you did that first Google search of Bell's: a lot of gruesome images. Most of the twisted faces you'll see on the Internet are of people at their worst in the first few weeks. You don't get before and after photos with most of them, although you can seek some out.

Many people have documented the stages of their condition on YouTube and other sites. This documentation could help if it makes you feel better, but I'm not one to recommend you place your private medical issues on the Internet for all to see for eternity. If you're just looking at others, don't let them scare you, and don't use their experience as a baseline for your own progress. Everyone heals differently. You might be one of the lucky ones and this whole thing could be behind you in a matter of weeks; or with all honesty, this could be a lifelong struggle. Many fall somewhere in the middle. Work at your recovery.

Here are some critical areas of treatment:

Warm Compresses
Massage, Acupuncture, Chiropractic
Vitamins & Protein
Food and drink
Exercises
Eye care
Social and psychological support

Let me define all of these options and provide my personal reactions:

Warm Compresses

One of the easiest but most important self-treatments was a warm washcloth on my face at night and whenever I could make the time during the day. Get the cloth hot, wring it out, and press firmly on your face. Move your fingers around and massage. Pretend you are playing a guitar on your face. Mimic a spider walking across your face. Let your face soak in the heat. Repeat a second or third time while lying down to relax. Do this 2-3 times a day or more, even in the shower, but especially at the end of the day just before going to sleep. Take this time to meditate. This relaxation is key to your recovery.

Massage

This is part of the long-term plan to keep those face muscles working and to keep the whole body relaxed. I started with face and head massages and then moved to full-body massages for relaxation. The face massage will hurt, but you will feel super upon finishing, and this treatment really does help keep the facial muscles alive and well. Most health centers that offer massage will offer face massage and have a therapist on staff familiar with the disorder. You could also seek out a specialist for sacral therapy. Most massage therapists at chain spas like *Hand and Stone* or *Massage Envy* are not entirely familiar with the disorder, but they can still help.

Full-body massage is great for everyone all the time. Some believe everyone should get a monthly massage. For this disorder, go as much as you can. Everything you do to relax your whole body will help your recovery. If you have a loved one in your home, ask if they would touch your face. They might be hesitant or afraid they're going to hurt you, but assure them that even the gentlest touch is not only going to feel great on that area, but it will actually assist in healing the area.

Acupuncture

I tried multiple sessions of acupuncture. The acupuncturist pokes your face and neck with needles, hooks up stimulation plugs, and turns on a low flow of electric to stimulate the facial muscles. None of this usually hurts, though the electric stimulation gets uncomfortable if it's set on too high. Be sure you let them know your comfort level before they walk away to let the stimulation do its job for thirty minutes or so. Even though my results were not significant and the financial cost was high, it was still worth it to include in my overall treatment. If I had been able to afford more sessions, I might have had better effects.

Some have reported better effects from a more aggressive acupuncture regimen. Studies in Asia, where acupuncture is widely used and more accepted have reported some benefits for Bell's Palsy. But those studies used an incredible number of treatment sessions, which is not financially feasible for most people in the Western world where virtually no insurance covers acupuncture.

Budget yourself between $80-125 per session. If you have the funds, then go for it. If not, fit this treatment in where you can.

Chiropractic

Many assume chiropractic adjustments are only useful for back and neck problems, but this treatment is great for your whole body. Have you had a toothache but found out the pain was really coming from a different tooth than the one you suspected? Have you had a neck pain and then found out it was really stemming from somewhere along your spinal column? People with spinal problems often feel pain in other various parts of the body including their neck, arms, hips, legs, and feet. They also suffer from headaches and anxiety. A spinal adjustment puts your bone structure back in balance, but it also solves pinched nerves and other nervous system and muscular issues.

Although sometimes people with severe neck and back problems will feel immediate relief, many will not. Those folks will see the effects a day or two later. You have to give chiropractic a chance to work.

If you're on a budget, there are now franchise chains where you can pop in for a quick adjustment at a good price, but be sure you check reviews or get a recommendation for a particular doctor. For a more comprehensive treatment, seek out a private chiropractor. They will spend more time with you and will incorporate additional treatment options like electrical stimulation, roller tables, and physical exercises. Unlike acupuncture, chiropractic is now covered by some insurance companies in the western world, but there may still be significant copays.

Even though chiropractic care has been shown to be effective in reducing symptoms in many patients, it is not a widely promoted treatment for Bell's Palsy. Like acupuncture, one could point to the varying number of months different patients will need to recover. Whether chiropractic treatment had anything to do with healing is not verifiable; perhaps they would've been at the same exact level of recovery. But anything that *could* help is worth a try, and the treatment could make you feel better in other ways by balancing out a body you didn't even know was out of alignment.

One weekly visit helped relax and balance me. I recommend anything that aids your overall health in any way, and chiropractic is a whole-body treatment that helps balance your structure and speed up recovery. You'll need everything you can to beat this Bell's.

Vitamins

The B vitamins are critical to the nervous system. Taking B6 and B12 vitamins may boost your recovery. I found an affordable bottle of B12 at *Target*. A dose is one tiny cherry flavored tablet each day for a blast of 100,000% the recommended value.

I also took 500-1,500 mg of vitamin C through chewable tablets found at my local *Trader Joes*. Vitamin C is essential for immune system defense and high mega-doses are often used around the world as part of the recovery process for many diseases. If you are in the U.S. you'll have to seek out a doctor who will administer pharmacologic levels of intravenous vitamin C. Many doctors won't offer it unless you inquire and insist.

Vitamin D is also important. While a deficiency hasn't been found to cause the problems, just about every person with every illness, including Bell's, has an identified vitamin D deficiency. You could take a D supplement, which would be recommended by your doctor if blood work reveals a deficiency, but many foods are fortified with D. Getting a bit of sunlight is also a great way to get your D for free.

I take a high-quality multi-vitamin, which happens to have D and a bit of C in it too. My intake of these multivitamins had lapsed for quite some time when I developed my own case of Bell's, so the diagnosis prompted me to get back to a quality multi-vitamin.

Selenium tablets, elderberry capsules, and turmeric capsules were also part of my daily supplement intake to help boost the immune system and fight inflammation. Dr. Neal Barnard also recommends the following for nerve damage: 600 milligrams a day of alpha-lipoic acid; 480 milligrams a day of gamma-linolenic acid and omega fatty acid; 1,000 milligrams a day of carnitine.

Protein

As with any medical recovery, getting a boost of protein will speed up the process. Even your dental surgeon will recommend a higher intake of protein after a dental extraction or implant.

My go to is *Vega* protein shakes, which pack 21 grams of plant protein without the negative effects that animal-based proteins leave you with such as saturated fat and high cholesterol. This vegan, gluten free, all natural pea protein goes pound for pound with any meat protein any day. It also contains a good amount of vitamin K and iron. I mix the chocolate or vanilla flavor mix (which is essentially void of sugar, only containing 1 gram) with a healthy vitamin D enriched rice milk drink in a tall glass once per day. I take my cherry flavored B-12 vitamin with it!

Food and Drink

The founder of modern medicine Hippocrates once exclaimed: "Food is thy Medicine"

As always, drink lots of clean water and eat lots of fresh organic fruits, vegetables, and whole grains. Animal fats found in meat are not beneficial to the nervous system or any system. Meat and dairy products have been found to promote inflammation, which is exactly what you want to avoid. I was saddened to find recommendations for those in a book for Bell's Palsy healing. So many nutritional studies now exist that confirm what we have known for a long time: a diet of meat and fats will make you sicker, while a plant-based diet will help you heal. If you don't believe me, read the numerous books and medical papers by Dr. John McDougall, Dr. Dean Ornish, Dr.

Caldwell Esselstyn, Dr. Neil Barnard, Dr. T. Colin Campbell, Dr. Brooke Goldner, Dr. Angie Sadeghi, and so many experts who testify to the health power of a plant-based diet.

More greens and grains will increase your fiber; this along with more fresh water will flush your body clean and lower your cholesterol, which is the best thing you can do for your cardiovascular and nervous systems. No single diet is going to heal your Bell's, but a more natural plant-based diet will support a whole-body healing during your recovery. You need to stack the deck in your favor.

Facial Exercises

These are not as important early on. In fact, you don't want to force your face muscles around too much because it runs the risk of synkinesis, which leaves people with uneven facial symmetry and twitches. This is what happens when the nerves reattach in the wrong places. I wouldn't recommend pushing your face too much until you feel like it's ready. The muscles are in shock and need to recuperate. Massage is the way to go early on.

But when you are ready, the exercises are as simple as raising the affected eyelid up and down. You'll need to assist the lift with your finger, but that's all right. Do the same with your smile by placing your finger at the corner of your mouth on the affected side, like the woman below. Note the three individuals on this book cover holding their smiles into position with their fingers. This smile lift is the only way you'll see your smile the way it was.

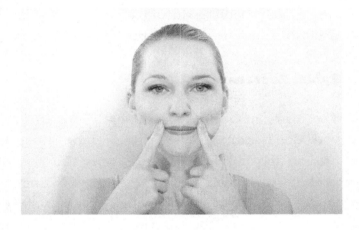

After speaking to so many victims of Bell's, I know the smile lift is a common practice for us, not just to revisit our old smile, but to actually exercise it. Move your lips and cheeks around! It's good for the muscles and nerves. Lift the paralyzed side up, to the side, and up again as you smile. Squint both of your eyes closed. You don't want to work the affected side without the other. What you want to do is train your face to move together again. When one side goes up, push the other side up.

Other movements you can practice are whistling, blowing bubbles, speaking, singing, blinking, and moving your lips side to side like the woman in the photo below.

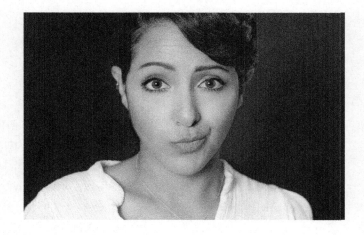

Honestly, these simple exercises may not come easy at first. Work at it and they will start to open up to you. You can find many free exercise resources on YouTube and the Internet, or you can attend a session or two with a physical therapist who will teach you what exercises to do on your own. There is nothing fancy about these exercises. These are common sense, so don't get roped into expensive weekly visits with a therapist unless there's a valid and thoroughly explained reason later in your recovery. Again, save this for later (3+ months), after giving your face some time to recuperate. Whether you work on your own or with a professional, physical therapy can be important in recovering those facial movements when the nerve is ready and able.

The Eye

Protecting your eye on the affected side is crucial from day one. My neurologist made the point that the single biggest thing to worry about with Bell's Palsy is the care of the eye. In the early days after onset, the eye will not be able to fully close in most cases. In the old days, doctors would send you home with a patch to protect the eye from damage while you sleep. These days it's all in the eye drops.

Your primary doctor should recommend a visit to an ophthalmologist. They will examine the eye carefully if you've had Bell's for some time before coming in to be sure no damage has been done. They will also want to see you back within weeks to be sure the eye is still being protected. An important point to remember: keep your eye lubricated with a general eye drop. Most will not assign a patch anymore because it's been found that the darkness and moisture do not help.

The affected eye will probably tear from the inability to blink. It's a strange sensation, but it will not last too long. Keep putting drops in during the day and then some thicker nighttime drops before bed. I used basic *ClearEye* during the day and *Systane* at night. You'll want to be sure you're going right to sleep after taking the nighttime drops because they will blur your eye; don't worry, you'll wake up clear eyed. Expect to use the eye drops and make bi-monthly visits for eye care for the first year even after your eye begins to blink again. I used the drops for about seven months straight to deal with the dry and strained eye. Many recoveries will be much quicker.

Wearing glasses during the day will be to your advantage. Get a vanity pair if you don't wear prescription glasses. Not only will the glasses protect your eye, but they will also serve as a distraction from your new face ailment. Because you'll find yourself very sensitive to light in the one eye, sunglasses will be essential to protect yourself from the sun and bright lights.

Social and Psychological Support

Find someone else who has or has had Bell's Palsy. This will change your entire outlook and make you feel better. Local support groups are going to be difficult to find in smaller cities, towns, and rural areas, but the magic of the Internet can connect you to hundreds of folks willing to help. Do a search on Twitter and Facebook and you'll be surprised at how many are out there. Finding someone else who has gone through this will have tremendous benefits of social support. I was fortunate to have a brother in law who had contracted Bell's only a year prior to mine. Andy and I live in different cities, but he was right there for me on my phone and late night texts.

If you are struggling to find someone or maintain a support system or are starting to feel really down on yourself, don't wait. Contact a professional therapist or psychologist. Talk to your primary doctor if need be. You don't have to go through anything alone. There are people out there willing to help and be there for you. Although you may feel alone and may feel that nobody understands you, don't isolate yourself. The quicker you get out and talk to friends or a professional, the better you'll feel.

If you are a parent or loved one reading this, look after your loved one. They may be feeling invisible and helpless. They need the support. There have been Bell's Palsy victims who had previously had cancer and claim they were more emotionally devastated by the palsy. Bell's Palsy has led to body dysmorphic disorder, depression, and suicide attempts, so do not take the effects of this lightly. On the other hand, know that this is a mostly temporary and physically harmless disorder.

Positivity

There are some theories out there that Bell's Palsy is really a symptom of stress, great stress. While there is a correlation, there is no proof of direct causation. But consider this: when your body and mind are under great stress, your immune system is going to be compromised, which makes you more prone to any illness. If Bell's Palsy is the result of damage due to viral activity the way we think it is, then your body will not have the resources to fight off the virus if your system is already stressed. This immune theory might also play into who bounces back quicker from the ailment versus someone who suffers with lingering effects. A positive frame of mind will undoubtedly help you through this disorder. So be social and talk to people, exercise, pray or meditate, and gets lots of great sleep— one of my favorite things to do in the early days of my Bell's. All of these will help relieve stress.

Watch a comedy film or show. You may need to hold your face if it hurts, but you need to feel that laughter and a smile forcing itself out. Laughter is healthy for you. It increases the endorphins released from your brain and relieves body tension. Laughter has also been found to ease pain, boost your immune system, burn calories, and protect the heart. Multiple studies show that laughter is one key trait in those who have the longest life spans. The benefits of laughter and smiling are enormous. Dopamine, endorphins, and serotonin are all released when you smile, which is why you need to work at getting back your smile as soon as possible and stay mentally healthy while you heal.

Other Considerations

Among some effective treatments found in early studies are hyperbaric oxygen therapy, Neuro-proprioceptive rehabilitation, EMG, mirror biofeedback, and mime therapy. Moxibustion is a heat therapy quite popular in Chinese traditional medicine often used in conjunction with acupuncture. Cold laser therapy is another new option. All of these are going to be difficult to track down, depending on where you live. Most physicians will have no expertise or knowledge in these approaches. Check for these treatments in a Google search to see if there are practitioners in or near your city who are able to help. I was not afforded the opportunity to try these, but if you want to heal, find your way. It's going to take some work and your own personalized plan.

For those with persisting issues, it may take longer. Botulinum toxin injections have been found to be useful for recurring spasms, according to Dr. Heckman. There are also surgical options with mixed results. Over 60% of the studies in one meta-analysis by Roy et al. showed some kind of complication. A more recent survey by Van Veen et al. showed good voluntary smiling ability for more patients following smile reanimation surgery. Opting for surgery should be your last resort.

There has been some controversial debate through the years over the use of antiviral treatment at diagnosis. Dr. Peter Kennedy reviewed older studies that brought up doubts about the success of the antivirals. One study found treatment with just the prednisolone steroid was slightly better than the steroid and anti-viral together. Another study showed no difference in recovery between patients who received the anti-viral valaciclovir and ones who did not. However, Kennedy also pointed to more newer studies that showed success of the antiviral combined with the steroid, and he called for further research concluding that he believed that "antiviral agents may have a role in treating severe cases of Bell's Palsy..." Don't worry about these debates right now. Get that rag on your face and finish your prescriptions.

Possibility is enough for me. A ten-day prescription of the anti-viral and steroid will not hurt you, even if they later find you have a different disorder. But if you do have Bell's Palsy, those two prescriptions are now believed to be essential in beginning your recovery.

If it's too late for you and you're past the first few days, don't fret. We went centuries without modern medicine and many still healed. Your recovery might be slower or incomplete, which is why you will want to rely on many of the varied approaches detailed in this chapter. Do all you can. As they say, throw everything and the kitchen sink at this.

Recovery

Recovery can be subjective in different degrees. Some reports predict just 2-3 weeks of recovery for the lucky select few. Most reports show recovery in 3-6 months. A minority of patients will wait up to a year to see recovery. As already mentioned, for victims who struggle to recover beyond a year or two, there are surgical and facial nerve decompression options as a last resort. The research says most recover fully with 90-100% of their original face.

A very small percentage of people will never get their original face back. An even smaller percentage have a more serious underlying issue like a brain tumor, but those are not genuine Bell's Palsy cases that occur suddenly overnight. Remember, if all you have is Bell's

Palsy, consider yourself fortunate because it's not dangerous, but let's also be honest: your face may never feel the way it did before this.

Risk Factors

It is important for everyone with Bell's Palsy to go through the needed evaluation and tests to rule out other disorders. Doctors Keels, Long, and Vann argue:

> Though a small percentage of children presenting with facial nerve paralysis have a brain stem tumor, a thorough medical evaluation is necessary to verify the absence of other neurological signs and symptoms which may reflect intracranial pathology. Bell's palsy should be a diagnosis of exclusion.

You need to rule out other conditions. Lyme disease, Guillain-Barre syndrome, Melkersson-Rosenthal syndrome, Ramsay Hunt syndrome, and cancer are other conditions sometimes misdiagnosed as Bell's Palsy, and all need immediate and specialized treatment. Once you have safely established that what you have is true Bell's Palsy, most of the physical health worries are gone and you are left with the social-emotional challenges.

There are a few final risk factors you should be aware of though:

- A study by Tseng et al. found a direct connection to increased anxiety in people who have or have recovered from Bell's Palsy.

- With a reoccurrence rate of about 12% (between 5 and 10% by some reports), one study reported up to 10% of patients afflicted will experience symptomatic recurrence after 10 years.

- One report by Warner et al. detailed possible eye complications as "corneal dryness leading to visual loss." The eye, yes, the eye, was my doctor's biggest concern.

- The previous report also warned of permanent damage to the facial nerve, and abnormal growth of nerve fibers.

- Some studies cited by Chiu et al. have shown Bell's Palsy patients are more likely to have a stroke later on.

Not exactly what you want to hear!

But my honesty is only to get you thinking about how you can minimize those risks. In dealing with the final risk of stroke, remember that diet, exercise, and more frequent and aggressive medical evaluations can save your life. Be vigilant and relentless in your fight to recovery. It's a long road.

Most of the healing approaches in this chapter are also productive ways of decreasing stress. In many ways, you will come out of this ailment just as strong, just as healthy, just as relaxed, and just as grateful for a second chance to smile.

In review, here are the key essentials you just can't do without if you are going to fight this disease and take back your smile:

Warm compresses
Massage
Healthy food and drink
Exercise
Eye care
Social and psychological support

SMILE IF YOU GOT ONE

On the night of January 13, 2019, I took to the mirror for a shave, and my life would never be the same. Stretching my face to get the razor into the crevice between my upper and lower lips, a painful cramp ripped through my jaw and neck— Oh my forties!

The pain subsided and I finished up. Only a minor passing muscle spasm on my cheek about a half hour later reminded me of the incident. I went to sleep and all seemed well.

When I woke up the next day, I went downstairs like every other morning, made my breakfast, and started to eat. That's when I realized my lips were not keeping the oatmeal in my mouth. The same with the pineapple juice. The waterfall of juice poured out like a hole in my lip. I went to the mirror to find my face was slightly crooked. The left side of my face was normal, but the right side was frozen. When I tried my hardest to raise an eyebrow or smile, nothing happened. It was like someone had cut a wire connecting my brain to that side of my face. Half my face was dead.

Remember the crooked, punkish, upper lip Billy Idol popularized in the 1980s? The "Rebel Yell" smile was roughly the only facial expression I was now capable of.

Soon enough, I was confident that I wasn't having a stroke because the rest of the right side of my body was working fine (and after several hours I was still alive). I walked around for the rest of the day avoiding social interaction, slurring my words when I was forced to speak, and struggling through meals. The next morning the physician's assistant confirmed my Google diagnosis of Bell's Palsy, a mysterious condition that usually paralyzes one side of the face and thankfully only one side, at least most of the time.

The condition, named after 19th century Scottish doctor Charles Bell, strikes 1 in 65 (about 40,000) Americans every year. There are 43 muscles in the face—43— exactly how old I was about to turn that year. But the muscles are not to blame. Without nerves, your muscles won't do much of anything. Bell's Palsy is due to inflammation of the seventh cranial nerve, which doctors believe is caused by injury or suspected virus. No doctor has yet to confirm whether it was the shaving injury, but I tend to think that was the moment.

It was Monday morning, so I had a class to teach at the university. I showed up and explained to the students that I had suffered an injury. I told them something vaguely about how the doctors were still looking into the remedy. Students stared and looked away, as I slurred through a quick lesson before setting them free to work in groups on a project. Is he drunk? Is he tired? Is he having a stroke? I imagined the internal questions drifting through the silent and polite room that day.

For the next several days, I read articles by other people, including fellow professors and public speakers, on how they coped with this condition. On the Internet, I viewed terrible images of people's twisted faces with cases far worse than my own. I combed the scholarly databases for professional opinions and studies. I realized it's an awful condition with unknown origins and the potential to derail a career, send mental health straight into decline, and upend a personal and social life.

There are many things we can do to prevent illness like eat our vegetables, take vitamins, exercise, avoid alcohol and tobacco, but sometimes we're still going to get hit with unpreventable disease, disorder, or injuries. Bell's Palsy can strike anyone, even the healthiest, and the worst part is it doesn't even have a confirmed cause. Scientists know what it is (the inflammation of the nerve) but they can't confirm what causes the inflammation. An awakened dormant virus is one popular theory. Somehow I don't think they'll honor my shaving injury as a possibility.

By the end of that first week, I was no better. My condition seemed to get slightly worse but it's possible it only felt this way due to my growing frustration as the days passed. I adapted as best as possible as the weeks passed. Some victims recover within two or three weeks. I was not in this lucky group. Other reports say three to six months. The research says most recover fully with 90-100% of their original face. But then there's a small percentage, perhaps those with far more extreme facial twisting than my damaged face, who never get their original face back.

Your face is far more than just vanity. A person's face shows life and death. Although a smile is not absolute evidence of accurate feelings, facial expressions are behavioral cues. Just think about all the functions your face muscles lend themselves to.

Consider all of the following obstacles caused by this disorder—

In the first several weeks, I had to relearn how to eat and drink, and even lost a few pounds (not such a bad side effect).

I had to work on my speech since I now talked out of one side of my mouth. I talked softer and less (not a bad effect for others). Any kind of speech impediment is a struggle in my line of work as a professor, but my students were supportive. To save my vocal energy for work, my regularly long phone talks with old friends were sadly postponed. Naturally, book events and workshops were canceled. Life was on pause.

In the fifth week, I attempted to project my voice a little more than needed out of the one side and I developed laryngitis for several days. Lesson learned.

Singing in the car was limited to Willie Nelson style— not a bad thing, just not what I was used to. But just listening to music was a struggle, since the ear on the affected side was hypersensitive to high pitch sounds. Since the seventh cranial nerve connects to your middle ear, severe ringing and strange echoes can last for months. So I opted for mostly silence for the first few weeks.

My right eye was unable to fully close and drained a load of tears down my cheek several times a day. I was extra sensitive to light and had to wear sunglasses more than usual, even indoors at times.

Months into this ordeal, I was still unable to whistle, which for most people might not be a big deal, but I was a real whistler. I would whistle in the car, on the street, in highs and lows, intricate classical based compositions, heavy metal solos, catchy pop riffs, all silenced now and stuck in my head.

My son needed to take the reins on blowing bubbles in the yard. I could not blow a simple bubble for months.

And blowing out the candles on my birthday cake later in the year seemed like it was going to be an impossible task.

But the worst part was my absent smile. A blank face. The puzzled looks I encountered when people couldn't read me. I was physically unable to express anything through my face, except for the twisted Rebel Yell.

Anyone who knows me knows I am usually quite the smiley fellow. I always have been. In school, it got me into trouble because teachers mistook it for wiseguy sarcasm, something mischievous, when all it was just a kid smiling and trying to make the best of life. A smile does not equate happiness though. For me smiling more was a way of trying to be happier, and while it doesn't work all of the time, it does work some of the time. One smile breeds other smiles, so you're likely to get a smile or two back in return, most of the time. Sometimes miserable people scoff at smiles.

I can remember one miserable woman at a store I worked at in New York when I was sixteen, who asked me with a huff, "Why are you always smiling?"

I remember at the time thinking,

"Because I'm not going to be working here much longer with you."

Maybe some people are being punished from a previous life and their smiles are restricted in this one. Maybe some lost the privilege. Maybe some never learned how. I'm not sure.

I began to wonder if smiles were regulated by some higher force. Maybe there is a limit on smiles. Maybe we only get two or three a day. Add in a few extra on holidays. That would be about 1,109 smiles a year, tops. If you live to eighty, that's about 88,720 allotted smiles!

But then look at the extremist with twenty-five or so smiles a day. That would amount to 9,125 a year. By the time they're in their early forties, they would have used up over 383,250 smiles. If they were a real joker, they could break a million smiles by age eighty-five. Those kinds of numbers could be considered abusive, by both the gods and damaged full-time store clerks. Maybe they see those kinds of numbers as demeaning. Maybe it just burns them inside to see someone else looking so damn happy. So they invented Bell's Palsy to prevent those kinds of numbers.

If I used up five to seven a day and maxed out in my forty-second year, that would mean the maximum allowed lifetime number of smiles would probably be somewhere around 90,000. Anything after that and Bell's Palsy kicks in.

But then how does my smile theory explain my inability to also frown? I was blank. Some people with Bell's have a noticeable droop in their face, which tells a stranger that there's probably a medical condition. But me? No, I was stuck with a normal looking straight face that made me look apathetic. My disability was under the skin.

Maybe it's better, I thought. Maybe I'd be taken more seriously with no facial expression. Maybe I'd get a huge promotion or become a CEO. Maybe I'd be welcomed into the ranks of the expressionless army.

My expressionless self gave no indication of what I was thinking. My blankness puzzled people, and I could tell the awkward moment when I lost someone. I had to rely on words. I had to explain, but at the same time I had to talk softer and say less, and it was all just so exhausting. Sometimes I didn't want to go there and explain anything. Sometimes I had to jump in with the difficult explanation of my condition to prevent offending someone. I had to pick my battles.

My wife had it worse than me. She was suddenly living with a stranger who she did not recognize. I had to explain with a straight face "It's me! It's me! I'm still in here." Her patience was remarkable.

Somehow my four and half-year-old son still looked in my eyes and knew when I was smiling. Most everyone else has had to do a double-take. I told him "Daddy has a boo-boo on his face. My smile will be back, but the doctor says it's going to take some time." I'm amazed that he understood this as a simple medical issue, when I was left questioning the cause in my logical and educated adult mind:

Is it voodoo?

A hex for speaking out on social issues?

Did I anger the gods?

Did I use up all of my smiles in this life?

The shaving explanation is still better than those.

It was an agonizing early arrival and ensuing philosophical dilemma in the parking lot as I contemplated whether this was "the end." I had waited over a month for the appointment. After the parking lot, it was onto a packed waiting room, a collection of sad stories, of the old and the young, and middle aged little me sitting in the middle of a room full of severe incurable neurological issues.

A very small percentage of people with Bell's symptoms have a more serious underlying issue like a brain tumor. That's not Bell's Palsy. Usually, those horrors develop slowly and do not suddenly appear overnight like Bell's Palsy. But you want to know for sure. The neurologist visit seemed like a verdict was about to be read on my future.

My name was called and minutes later a nurse was asking me questions. These were the same answers I repeated to multiple doctors for weeks. Others told me there would be a barrage of more intense tests this time. Yet when the neurologist arrived, a handshake was the extent of our contact. He didn't order any new tests. He barely smiled.

A dentist had previously hoodwinked me into a $400 CT scan, which the neurologist chuckled at and told me to keep when I offered to share it. I had suspected a dental issue, and my obviously wrong suspicion cost me. For another $80, an ear, nose, and throat specialist gave me the nod for no ENT issues.

The neurologist also charged me an $80 copay to give me a Google answer and to share his supreme confidence that I would survive. He confirmed what I already knew from Google— it's going to take some time to get my smile back, and apparently some money too.

After my primary doctor listened to my concerns in a follow-up visit, as he always does (I am very fortunate for this), he gave me referrals to occupational and physical therapists and an ophthalmologist. He smiled at my shaving theory and approved of my "alternative" attempts to manage the problem. Chiropractic visits were already underway. Acupuncture too. And massage was a godsend! I was going to be busy treating this for a while.

The months went on during the spring semester of 2019. I started bringing a smiley-face mask to class and would hold it up in front of my face every time I wanted to smile. The disorder made me a little funnier.

I desperately looked forward to sleep every night, since I felt it was an escape from my new reality. I hoped I'd wake and find it had all been a bad dream and that my smile was restored in the morning. But I only woke up every morning disappointed and sometimes even in fear that the little progress I had made would all be erased by a recurrence.

I read about movie stars and newscasters who had been struck with the condition, and I had sympathy for them knowing how important their face is, but I also scoffed at the stories of their terrible two weeks before a full recovery. I would be months away.

By May of 2019, I found my face back at what I considered 75-80%. Not bad. I'll take what I can get.

Now almost two years later, while I can smile again, it is not what it was. I do not have full flexibility, and social interaction can be challenging. I have learned how to position myself at the right angle so when someone meets me they're looking at my better side. For photographs, I learned to turn to the side. Worse though is when I laugh or smile too hard, which sends me into a hand-clenching charley horse that rips through my jaw and cheek. I have to actually regulate my smiles and laughs.

Facial expressions are exhausting, which is why a very small percentage of the population including myself (and maybe even yourself) was oddly relieved when the COVID-19 pandemic struck. By spring of 2020, the rest of the world would join us in masks.

Social distancing? Great.
Masks? Even better.

The liberation of putting on that surgical facemask for the first time during the pandemic and heading out into a world where I wouldn't have to work to conceal my strange condition, knowing everyone (well, almost everyone) would be joining me in a faceless world. Perhaps only those who have awoken to the thief of smiles may understand this.

But take a moment and think about that time you found yourself smiling in public only to realize your protective mask was on and no one could see it. That's exactly how I felt for nearly five months. That's exactly how you probably feel right now, along with a million other people across the planet.

I'm very grateful. It could always be worse.

I'm going to fight for a full recovery. I don't care about the voodoo, or the hex, or the angry gods— I'm going to try my hardest to smile, even if it hurts.

BRIEF NOTE ON POST-COVID BELIEFS

With over 5 billion vaccinated against Covid, it's illogical to assert that the vaccine causes Bell's Palsy. If true, that would be a lot of people with facial palsy! But some people on the Internet have asserted that the Covid vaccine causes various diseases all at once, including blood clots, stroke, heart disease, and even cancer. It's peculiar that one vaccine causes so many different simultaneous diseases that have already existed for thousands of years. In fact, Bell's Palsy was documented over 2,500 years ago before modern chemicals and vaccines existed. Even though adults in their 30s and 40s are the prime population to get Bell's, they haven't had vaccines in quite some time. If the odd beliefs of "neurotoxins" and "vaccines" causing Bell's and other disorders were true, children who are our most recently vaccinated population would have record numbers of problems. Thankfully, this is not true.

It is a problem that the general public does not have access to the best and newest medical research published in the databases, but an even greater problem is their inability to properly interpret the few free articles published online. In 2020, someone posted a letter by three doctors, Colella et al., claiming it was evidence that the vaccine caused Bell's Palsy. The problems with the letter: 1. Their report was of just one person. 2. He was 37, the prime age for Bell's Palsy, 3. He wasn't tested for herpes simplex, 4. This was a letter, and not a peer reviewed research study, 5. The letter uses one study as evidence to support their suggestion, 6. That one study by Baden et al. reported just seven people with Bell's after getting vaccinated, 7. The doctors were understandably rushing to document what they considered could be an early case of something, which was of course soon refuted by multiple studies later published.

Another report available on the Internet was also circulated as belief for cause and effect. This report also featured just one patient. The one patient was 50 years old, again prime age for Bell's Palsy. The one patient developed Bell's three weeks after his second dose of the

Covid vaccine. All unconvincing to anyone who has studied the disease. The report writers Ish and Ish were decent enough to conclude that "the association may be a mere coincidence." But the Internet loves coincidences.

In one paper, Tamaki et al. disclosed how the FDA cited insufficient evidence to determine causal association between COVID vaccinations and Bell's Palsy, yet they cited two phase 3 COVID-19 vaccine trials as a reason for concern. The two trials consisted of 73,868 participants (36,930 were vaccinated) and Bell's Palsy was not even listed as a significant adverse event. Out of all those people, there were only 7 reported cases of Bell's Palsy.

One of the cited studies in the Tamaki et al paper, was Baden et al., which used 30,420 participants. Four patients ended up with Bell's Palsy, but only three were vaccinated, with the fourth in the placebo group. This amounts to <0.1% occurrence. Baden et al. called it anecdotal, yet also rang an alarm and suggested surveillance, oddly citing the second trial, which was cited by Tamaki et al. The second trial by Polack et al. doesn't even mention Bell's Palsy. We can certainly attribute some of the online fear to careless reporting.

Hysteria resulted from another Internet news story, where a very small number of people experienced mild facial palsy after the vaccine. *The Jerusalem Post* reported that the study included just 13 cases of facial palsy out of two million vaccinated. 1, 3, 30, or even 300 cases of Bell's Palsy are all statistically within the norm; in other words, it's a coincidence & these people would've gotten the disease anyway. With the number of people vaccinated, Bell's cases would need to be in the hundreds of thousands to be a concern.

On the contrary, getting the Covid virus if you're unvaccinated has been found to give you a slightly greater risk of contracting Bell's Palsy. But like the flawed vaccine beliefs, there are problems with claiming that this virus is a cause of Bell's. Many of those reports concerning the virus also use extremely small sample sizes of participants. Estakhr et al argued that there is reason to conclude that there is enough evidence to suggest that SARS-CoV-2 infection may cause facial nerve palsy, yet their study is based on just 36 participants. Codeluppi et al. found "about 21% of patients presenting to the emergency department for facial palsy during COVID-19 outbreak had active or recent symptoms consistent with COVID-19 infection" and concluded that there was a higher incidence of facial palsy during the pandemic based on only 38 patients. Gupa and Jawanda declared the possibility of a Covid cause for Bell's Palsy; their study featured only 46 patients. Islamoglu et al found that the SARS-CoV-2 IgM + IgG antibody test was positive in 24.3% of the patients with facial palsy; their study featured 41 patients. Another article by Yue Wan suggests Covid may be a cause of Bell's Palsy, yet only one patient in a case report was used to make this bold conclusion. Even with larger sample sizes, none of this proves a cause of Bell's Palsy.

One letter of concern from Tamaki et al. reviewed a massive number of 348,088 patients with the virus. 284 were diagnosed with Bell's Palsy within eight weeks of their Covid diagnosis. That small number amounts to just 0.08%. While 153 of the patients (53.9%) had no history of the disorder, an amazingly high number (131, 46.1%) had a history of Bell's Palsy. One point they had was that the unvaccinated Covid patients had a significantly elevated risk of Bell's Palsy compared to the vaccinated.

It seems every study shows little reason to be concerned with Bell's Palsy as compared to the valid side effects of Covid-19, yet a few have the need to raise a flag of concern, which could set off false alarms in the general public.

One final flaw about many of these reports concerning both the virus and vaccine is they only compare 2020 to the previous year. One year of comparison is hardly a fair and logical comparison. We have a hundred years of data in many places, and we know the numbers of Bell's Palsy patients have always fluctuated. For example, one year could produce 10 cases per 100,000. The very next year could be 50 per 100,000. Zammit et al. reported that the facial nerve palsy rate was 2.7% higher than last year, but their study was only six months, in only one city (Liverpool, with a small population of 498,00), and failed to compare to rates beyond the previous year of comparison. When looking further back, Shemer et al determined a stable trend from the number of cases for facial nerve palsy during the preceding years (2015-2020) and found no association between the vaccine and an increased risk of facial palsy.

FINAL ADVICE

While you are recovering your smile, you'll want to consider one more thing: how you handle social situations. Even in quarantine during a pandemic, you're likely to be expected to make a video appearance (without a mask on). So here's my best advice, much of which I picked up from a *New Yorker* magazine article written by New York professor and Bell's Palsy veteran Jonathan Kalb:

When smiling, turn your head away and down on a slight angle from the person so that your better side is pointing in their direction. You'll be moving your palsy side away from the person to create an illusion. You can practice this and variations of your smile in the mirror on a daily basis. Remember though that real emotions could push your face in directions you might not be preparing for in the mirror. This happens to me when I'm brought to a heavy laugh or when I'm in an environment when I'm smiling a lot to be friendly. Yes, you will actually get tired from smiling. You may also get an occasional Charley horse cramp in your face (not fun) when you smile too big. This smile business is real work. Take it easy and be well.

NOTE OF GRATITUDE

Whether you have just woken up with Bell's Palsy, or you've moved on and fully recovered, or you're entering another year with the remnants (like I am), or you're a curious and caring family member or friend of someone who has woken up with this awful condition, I sincerely hope this book has helped you. Thank you for reading, keep at it, and be safe.

All the best,
Bill

REFERENCES

Alp H, Tan H, Orbak Z. Bell's palsy as a possible complication of hepatitis B vaccination in a child. *J Health Popul Nutr.* 2009;27(5):707.

Akhtar A. The flaws and human harms of animal experimentation. *Camb Q Healthc Ethics.* 2015; 24(4):407-419.

Baden LR, El Sahly HM, Essink B, et al. Efficacy and Safety of the mRNA-1273 SARS-CoV-2 Vaccine. *N Engl J Med.* 2021;384(5):403-416. doi:10.1056/NEJMoa2035389

Barnard, N. *Dr. Neil Barnard's Program for Reversing Diabetes,* Rodale, 2017.

Bardage C, Persson I, Ortqvist A, Bergman U, Ludvigsson JF, Granath F. Neurological and autoimmune disorders after vaccination against pandemic influenza A (H1N1) with a monovalent adjuvanted vaccine: population based cohort study in Stockholm, Sweden. *BMJ.* 2011;343:d5956. Published 2011 Oct 12.

BBC News. Bell's palsy: 'I woke and the night had stolen my smile' 3 May 2019. www.bbc.com

Braus, Hermann- Anatomie des Menschen: ein Lehrbuch für Studierende und Ärzte 1921, Public Domain, commons.wikimedia.org

Cai Z, Li H, Wang X, Niu X, Ni P, Zhang W, Shao B. Prognostic factors of Bell's palsy and Ramsay Hunt syndrome. *Medicine.* 2017 Jan; 96(2):e58.

Chakravarti, A., Chaturvedi, V. N., Bhide, V., & Rodrigues, J. J. Bell's Palsy - herpes simplex virus type-1.... *Indian journal of otolaryngology and head and neck surgery. 1999; 51*(2), 47–50.

Chen JK. Bell's palsy from dental infection. Zhonghua Yi Xue Za Zhi. 1945;31(3-4):242-.

Chiu Y, Yen M, Chen L, et al. Increased risk of stroke after Bell's palsy: a population-based longitudinal study. *Journal of Neurology, Neurosurgery & Psychiatry* 2012; 83:341-343.

Codeluppi, L, Venturelli, F, Rossi, J, et al. Facial palsy during the COVID-19 pandemic. *Brain Behav*. 2021; 11:e01939. h̲

Colella G, Orlandi M, Cirillo N. Bell's palsy following COVID-19 vaccination. *J Neurol*. 2021;268(10).

Colledge L. Descendens Noni Facial Anastomosis for Bell's. *Proc R Soc Med*. 1927; 20(7):1138.

Cotton BA. Chiropractic care of a 47-year-old woman with chronic Bell's palsy: a case study. *J Chiropr Med*. 2011;10(4):288-293.

COVID-19 vaccine: 13 out of nearly 2 mil Israelis suffer facial paralysis. *Jerusalem Post*. Jan. 2021.
De Diego-Sastre JI, Prim-Espada MP, Fernández-García F. [The epidemiology of Bell's palsy]. *Rev Neurol*. 2005 Sep 1-15; 41(5): 287.

Drumm C. Can the COVID-19 vaccine cause Bell's palsy? experts say no. *The Health Nexus*. Jan. 2021.

Estakhr M, Tabrizi R, Ghotbi Z, Shahabi S, Habibzadeh A, Bashi A, Borhani-Haghighi A. Is facial nerve palsy an early manifestation of COVID-19? A literature review. *Am J Med Sci.* April 2022.

Facial Palsy. UK. 2020. www.facialpalsy.org

Finsterer, J., & Grisold, W. Disorders of the lower cranial nerves. *Journal of neurosciences in rural practice*, 2015; 6(3), 377–391.

Fu X, Tang L, Wang C, et al. A Network Meta-Analysis to Compare the Efficacy of Steroid and Antiviral Medications for Facial Paralysis from Bell´s Palsy. *Pain Physician.* 2018; 21(6):559-.

Gupta S, Jawanda MK. Surge of Bell's Palsy in the era of COVID-19: Systematic review. *Eur J Neurol.* 2022 Apr 28. doi: 10.1111/ene.15371.

Heckmann JG, Urban PP, Pitz S, Guntinas-Lichius O, Gágyor I: The diagnosis and treatment of idiopathic facial paresis (Bell's palsy). Dtsch Arztebl Int 2019; 116: 692–702.

Ish S, Ish P. Facial nerve palsy after COVID-19 vaccination - A rare association or a coincidence. *Indian J Ophthalmol.* 2021;69(9):2550

Islamoglu Y, Celik B, Kiris M. Facial paralysis as the only symptom of COVID-19: A prospective study. *Am J Otolaryngol.* 2021;42(4).

Kalb, Jonathan. Give me a smile. *The New Yorker.* January 2015.

Keels, Martha Ann & Long, L & Vann, William. Facial nerve paralysis: report of two cases of Bell's palsy. *Pediatric dentistry.* 1987; 9. 58.

Kennedy, P. Herpes simplex virus type 1 and Bell's palsy—a current assessment of the controversy. *Journal of NeuroVirology.* 2010;16.

Lamina, S., & Hanif, S. Pattern of facial palsy in a typical Nigerian specialist hospital. *African health sciences,* 2012; 12(4), 514–517.

Levine, Deena & Adelman, Mara. *Beyond Language: Cross Culture.* Prentice Hall, 1993.

Lima MA, Silva MTT, Soares CN, et al. Peripheral facial nerve palsy associated with COVID-19. *J Neurovirol.* 2020; 26(6):941-944.

Lynch, P.J. Brain in human normal inferior view. Medical illustrator derivative work: Beao, Brain human normal inferior view, *CC BY* 2.5

May M, Fria TJ, Blumenthal F, Curtin H: Facial paralysis in children: differential diagnosis. *Otolaryngol Head Neck Surg.*1981; 89: 841-48.

McCormick D. P. Herpes-simplex virus as a cause of Bell's palsy. *Lancet, 1 1972;* (7757), 937.

Murakami S, Mizobuchi M, Nakashiro Y, Doi T, Hato N, Yanagihara N. Bell palsy and herpes simplex virus: identification of viral DNA in endoneurial fluid and muscle. Ann Intern Med. 1996 Jan 1;124(1 Pt 1):27-30.

Mutsch M, Zhou W, Rhodes P, et al. Use of the inactivated intranasal influenza vaccine and the risk of Bell's. *N Engl J Med.* 2004; 350(9):896-.

Penn JW, James A, Khatib M, et al. Development and validation of a computerized model of smiling:

Modeling the percentage movement required for perception. *J Plast Reconstr Aesthet Surg.* 2013; 66(3):345-351.

Perusquía-Hernández M, Ayabe-Kanamura S, Suzuki K. Human perception and biosignal-based identification of posed and spontaneous smiles. *PLoS One.* 2019; 14(12):e0226328.

Polack FP, Thomas SJ, Kitchin N, et al. Safety and Efficacy of the BNT162b2 mRNA Covid-19 Vaccine. *N Engl J Med.* 2020;383(27):2603-2615. doi:10.1056/NEJMoa2034577

Pourmomeny, A. A., & Asadi, S. Management of synkinesis and asymmetry in facial nerve palsy: a review article. *Iranian journal of otorhinolaryngology,* 2014; 26(77), 251–256.

Pourrat, O., Neau, J. P., & Pierre, F. Bell's palsy in pregnancy: HELLP syndrome or pre-eclampsia? *Obstetric medicine,* 2013; 6(3), 132–.

Preuschoft, S. "Laughter" and "Smile" in Barbary Macaques, Macaca sylvanus. *Ethology,* 1992; 91: 220-236.

Reaves, E.J., Ramos, M. & Bausch, D.G. Workplace cluster of Bell's palsy in Lima, Peru. *BMC Res Notes* 2014; 7, 289.

Riga M, Kefalidis G, Danielides V The role of diabetes mellitus in the clinical presentation and prognosis of Bell palsy. *J Am Board Fam Med* 2012; 25:819–26

Roy M, Corkum JP, Shah PS, et al. Effectiveness and safety of the use of gracilis muscle for dynamic smile restoration in paralysis: *J Plast Reconstr Aesthet Surg*. 2019; 72(8):1254-1264.

Sajadi, M. M., Sajadi, M. R., & Tabatabaie, S. M. The history of facial palsy and spasm: Hippocrates to Razi. *Neurology*, 2011; 77(2).

Sanders R. D. The Trigeminal (V) and Facial (VII) Cranial Nerves: Head and Face Sensation and Movement. *Psychiatry*, 2010; 7(1), 13–16.

Santos, Mônica A. de Oliveira, C. Filho, H. Vianna, M. Ferreira, Almeida, & Lazarini. Varicella zoster virus in Bell's palsy. *Brazilian Journal of Otorhinolaryngology*, 2010; 76(3), 370.

Shemer A, Pras E, Einan-Lifshitz A, Dubinsky-Pertzov B, Hecht I. Association of COVID-19 Vaccination and Facial Nerve Palsy: A Case-Control Study. *JAMA Otolaryngol Head Neck Surg*. 2021;147(8):739–743. doi:10.1001/jamaoto.2021.1259

Skuladottir, A.T., Bjornsdottir, G., Thorleifsson, G. *et al.* A meta-analysis uncovers the first sequence variant conferring risk of Bell's palsy. *Sci Rep* 11, 4188 (2021).

Spillane JD. Bell's Palsy and Herpes Zoster. *Br Med J.* 1941;1(4180):236-237.

Sweeney, C. J., & Gilden, D. H. (2001). Ramsay Hunt syndrome. *Journal of neurology, neurosurgery, and psychiatry, 71*(2), 149–154.

Tamaki A, Cabrera CI, Li S, et al. Incidence of Bell Palsy in Patients With COVID-19. *JAMA Otolaryngol Head Neck Surg*. 2021;147(8):767–768.

Takahashi, H., Hitsumoto, Y., Honda, N., Hato, N., & al. Mouse model of bell's palsy induced by reactivation of herpes simplex virus type 1. *Journal of Neuropathology and Experimental Neurology, 2001; 60*(6), 621-7.

Thomas, W. Facial paralysis in animals. *Merck Vet Manual,* 2021. merckvetmanual.com
Jul 2021 | Content last modified Sep 2021

Trumble, Angus. *A Brief History of the Smile.* Basic Books, 2005.

Tseng, C. C., Hu, L. Y., Liu, M. E., Yang, A. C., Shen, C. C., & Tsai, S. J. Bidirectional association between Bell's palsy and anxiety disorders, *Journal of affective disorders,* 2017; 215, 269-.

Tseng HF, Sy LS, Ackerson BK, et al. Safety of Quadrivalent Meningococcal Conjugate Vaccine in 11 to 21 Year-Olds. *Pediatrics.* 2017;139(1).

van Veen MM, Dusseldorp JR, Quatela O, et al. Patient experience in nerve-to-masseter-driven smile reanimation. *J Plast Reconstr Aesthet Surg.* 2019; 72(8):1265-1271.

Varejão AS, Muñoz A, Lorenzo V. Magnetic resonance imaging of the intratemporal facial nerve in idiopathic facial paralysis in the dog. *Vet Radiol Ultrasound.* 2006 Jul-Aug;47(4):328-33.

Wald A, Corey L. Persistence in the population: epidemiology, transmission. In: Arvin A, Campadelli-Fiume G, Mocarski E, et al., editors. *Human Herpesviruses: Biology, Therapy, and Immunoprophylaxis.* Cambridge: Cambridge University Press; 2007. Chapter 36.

Warner MJ, Hutchison J, Varacallo M. Bell Palsy. [Updated 2020 Mar 24]. In: StatPearls [Internet]. Treasure Island (FL): StatPearls Publishing; 2020 Jan. Available from: www.ncbi.nlm.nih.gov

Yue Wan, Shugang Cao, Qi Fang et al. Coronavirus disease 2019 complicated with Bell's palsy: a case report, 16 April 2020.

Zammit, M. Markey, A. Webb, C.A rise in facial nerve palsies during the coronavirus disease 2019 pandemic. *J Laryngol Otol,* 134 (10) (2020), pp. 905.

Zhao H, Zhang X, Tang YD, Zhu J, Wang XH, Li ST. Bell's Palsy: Clinical Analysis of 372 Cases and Review of Related Literature. *Eur. Neurol.* 2017; 77(3-4):168-172.

FURTHER RESOURCES

Author's Note: I am not affiliated with any of the following organizations, but I encourage you to explore more resources on your own if you have the time. Of course, as warned in the beginning of this book, be cautious of the many web sources that lack credibility and attempt to sell the best new cure. Further exploration of legitimate organizations and clinics might be particularly useful should you be interested in becoming a part of a study or curious about trying a new form of treatment. Some will be free, but some will be costly. Oxygen therapy, for example, looks very promising, but it's difficult to find and very expensive. But don't stop looking. I know I won't. This has become a lifelong quest and I plan on periodically updating this book to reflect any new findings.

American Association of Neuromuscular & Electrodiagnostic Medicine
2621 Superior Drive NW
Rochester, MN 55901
507.288.0100
aanem@aanem.org
www.aanem.org

Ask Doctor Jo
Doctor Jo is a physical therapist who shares excellent facial exercises for Bell's Palsy. You can find her video on Youtube or her website.
www.askdoctorjo.com

Brain Resources and Information Network (BRAIN)
Bethesda, MD 20824
800-352-9424

Crystal Touch Bell's Palsy Clinic
The Netherlands
https://crystal-touch.nl/
info@crystal-touch.nl

Facial Palsy UK
Telephone enquiries: 0300 030 9333
info@facialpalsy.org.uk

National Library of Medicine
National Institutes of Health/DHHS
Bethesda, MD 20894
888-346-3656
www.nlm.nih.gov

National Organization for Rare Disorders
55 Kenosia Avenue
Danbury, CT 06810
orphan@rarediseases.org
800-999-NORD (6673)

Sir Charles Bell Society
www.sircharlesbell.com

ABOUT THE AUTHOR

Dr. William K. Lawrence teaches research and science writing at NC State University in Raleigh, North Carolina in the United States. He is the author of ten books including *Learning and Personality, 89 Days,* and the novel *The Punk and the Professor.*

Printed in Great Britain
by Amazon